Cauterization in Traditional System of Medicine

(Electrocautery)

By

Kalpna Ijm (MD)

Rajiv Gandhi University, Bangalore

India

CS Independent Publishing Platform, South Carolina, North Charleston, USA

Book Details

Paperback: 74 pages
Publisher: CS Independent Publishing Platform; 2nd edition (April, 2016)
Language: English
ISBN-10: **1530920760**
ISBN-13: **978-1530920761**
Product Dimensions: 6 x 9 inches

Corresponding email: kalpnajanardan@gmail.com

Cauterization in traditional system of medicine
First Edition: 2014, Second Ed 2016
Publisher: CS Independent Publishing Platform; 2nd edition

Notice

Kalpna Ijm

About the book

Cauterization is an ancient medical procedure, now days comprises of electrocautery, and chemical cautery commonly. The evidence of use of cauterization for remove an undesired growth, or minimize other potential medical harmful possibilities such as infections, when antibiotics are not available procedure can be traced back in ancient system of medicine like Greco-roman, Indian and Arabic medicine. In early of 19th century their uses were very common among European surgeons for the means of natural and cosmetic healing in superficial and other surgical cut. Now a days cauterization is an established therapeutic modality among Indian system of medicine (*Unani*). It is being commonly used to remove benign lesions on the surface of the skin such as warts, skin tags and seborrheic keratosis. In this book author comprises the possible indications of cauterization along with procedures, safety concerns, historical perspective, surgical

4

operative standards, and contraindication of the same described in *traditional* system of medicine.

This book is doctor-friendly because it would help the alternative medical practitioners involved in providing not only curative services, but also preventive and promotive services to the community at large, motivating them to a healthier, and happier life.

Despite my sincere efforts to make the book accurate and comprehensive as i could, it is possible there may be some gaps or errors in the book. I would be most grateful to the readers, if these deficiencies are pointed out so that can be removed in the next edition. I also invite healthy suggestions from all readers to help me improve the quality of book and achieve the purpose with which it has been written. All such feedback would be carefully considered and gratefully acknowledged.

Kalpna Ijm

Skin is the largest and the first noticeable organ of your body. It is your skin, which captures everyone's attention. Get rid of all your skin ailments and feel beautiful!

"You are beautiful, when you make your skin comfortable"

INDEX

CAUTERIZATION

Cauterization

The medical practice or technique of cauterization is a medical term describing the burning of part of a body to remove or close off a part of it in a process called cautery, which destroys some tissue, in an attempt to mitigate damage, remove an undesired growth, or minimize other potential medical harmful possibilities such as infections, when antibiotics are not available. The practice was once widespread and is still used in remote regions of the world such as central Australia for treatment of wounds. Its utility before the advent of antibiotics was effective on several levels:

- ❖ Useful in stopping severe blood-loss,
- ❖ To close amputations,
- ❖ Useful in preventing infections, including complications from septicaemia.

Actual cautery is a term referring to the white-hot iron-a metal generally heated only up to a dull red glow—that is applied to produce blisters, to stop bleeding of a blood vessel, and other similar purposes.

The main forms of cauterization used today in the first world are electrocautery and chemical cautery—where both are, for example, prevalent in the removal of unsightly warts. Cautery can also mean the branding of a human, either recreational or forced. Accidental burns can be considered cauterization as well.

HISTORY

History of cauterization

Cauterization was used to stop heavy bleeding, especially during amputations. The procedure was simple: a piece of metal was heated over fire and applied to the wound. This would cause tissues and blood to heat rapidly to extreme temperatures in turn causing coagulation of the blood thus controlling the bleeding, at the cost of extensive tissue damage. The old fashioned form of cautery was a little··· less refined. A (typically iron) implement was heated to glowing red hot and pressed against or into an open wound, typically deeper wounds like arrow or bullet hole. In most cases, the person would have been better served to apply pressure to stop bleeding and then keep the wound clean with boiled water.

The other historical use for cautery is to seal a field amputation. Amputation is the removal of a whole or partial limb, typically arms, legs, feet, or toes (or more rarely, castration). Prior to modern micro-surgical technique (and especially in battle-field situations where time was limited and patient numbers were overwhelming) amputations were performed by applying a tourniquet above the cut line to prevent massive bleeding, cutting through the tissue to the bone, sawing through the bone, and cutting through the remaining tissue. As you can imagine, this was a very blood procedure. The risks of infection were astronomical, but the risks of bleeding to death when the tourniquet was removed were even higher. Rather than allow their patients to die from blood loss, field surgeons performed cautery to seal the end of the amputation. Keep in mind this was also before the use of anesthesia became widespread.

Cautery is described in the Hippocratic Corpus. The cautery was employed for almost every possible purpose in ancient times: as a 'counter-irritant', as a haemostatic, as a bloodless knife, as a means of destroying tumours, etc. Later, special medical instruments called cauters were used to cauterize arteries. These were first described by Abu al-Qasim al-Zahrawi (Abulcasis) in his *Kitab al-Tasrif*. Abu al-Qasim al-Zahrawi also introduced the technique of ligature of the arteries as an alternative to cauterization. This method was later improved and used more effectively by Ambroise Paré.

Differences Between Electrosurgery & Electrocautery

The terms electrosurgery and electrocautery are frequently confused, even amongst many professionals working in various healthcare related fields. And even though both of these procedures are applied within several medical specialties, they are quite different in terms of both tools used and method of application.

The Significant Differences

Let's take a closer look at both procedures in-order to further illustrate the differences between the two in terms of therapeutic application and the tools used.

1. Electrosurgery passes electrical current through tissue to accomplish a desired result. The electricity used is a form of alternating current similar to the that used

to generate radio waves. The typical frequency is quite high, with the norm being around 500, 000 cycles per second. This ensures that the current passes through the patients tissue as opposed to producing an electric shock effect. The heat is created by the resistance of the tissue to the electrical current and the tools used to apply the current are electrodes and includes blades, round ball, needle and loop configurations . The electrode selection depends upon and intended outcome.. These instruments can be used to cut, coagulate , or even to fuse tissue.

2. Electrocautery uses electrical current to heat a metal wire that is then applied to the target tissue in order to burn or coagulate the specific area of tissue. It is not used to pass the current through tissue, but rather is applied directly onto the targeted area of treatment. Using this technique, heat is passed through a resistant metal wire which is used as an electrode. This hot

electrode is then placed directly onto the treatment area destroying that specific tissue. This use of electricity is typically applied in superficial situations encountered by dermatologists, ophthalmologists, plastic surgeons, urologists, and related specialties.

3. Another rather obvious difference between the two is that electrocautery devices are usually small, battery operated, devices which use physical heat to destroy the targeted tissues or cause a specific and desired effect. The electosurgery devices are more sophisticated radio-wave generators that pass modified electrical current through the target tissues to achieve the desired surgical result.

The bottom line here is that *electrosurgery* is not synonymous with *electrocautery*, despite their mutual use of electrical current to deliver their respective treatment goals.

ELECTROCAUTERY

Electrocautery

Electrocauterization is the process of destroying tissue using heat conduction from a metal probe heated by electric current (much like a soldering iron). The procedure is used to stop bleeding from small vessels (larger vessels being ligated) or for cutting through soft tissue. Unlike electrocautery, electrosurgery is based on generation of heat inside tissue, using electric current passing through the tissue itself. Electrocautery is used in the treatment of skin cancers via electrodessication and curettage. Electrocauterization is preferable to chemical cauterization because chemicals can leach into neighbouring tissue and cauterize outside of the intended boundaries.

Electrocautery applies high frequency alternating current by a unipolar or bipolar method. It can be a continuous waveform to cut tissue, or intermittent to coagulate tissue. Ultrasonic coagulation and ablation systems are also available.

Unipolar

In unipolar cauterization, the physician contacts the tissue with a single small electrode. The circuit's exit point is a large surface area, such as the buttocks, to prevent electrical burns. The amount of heat generated depends on size of contact area, power setting or frequency of current, duration of application, and waveform. Constant waveform generates more heat than intermittent. Frequency used in cutting the tissue is higher than in coagulation mode.

Bipolar

Bipolar electrocautery passes the current between two tips of a forceps-like tool. It has the advantage of not disturbing other electrical body rhythms (such as the heart) and also coagulates tissue by pressure. Lateral thermal injury is greater in unipolar than bipolar devices.

Electrocauterization is preferable to chemical cauterization, because chemicals can leach into neighbouring tissue and cauterize outside of intended boundaries, Concern has also been raised regarding toxicity of the surgical smoke electrocautery produces. This contains chemicals that, through inhalation, may harm patients or medical staff.

In electrocautery, the current does not pass through the patient; thus, the procedure can be safely used in patients with implanted electrical devices such as cardiac pacemakers, implantable cardioverter-defibrillators, and deep-brain stimulators.

In contrast, electrosurgery is a group of commonly used procedures that utilize the passage of high-frequency alternating electrical current through living tissue to achieve varying degrees of tissue destruction. Different forms of electrosurgery include electrocoagulation, electrofulguration, electrodesiccation, and electrosection. Electrosurgery produces electromagnetic interference, which can interfere with implanted medical devices.

Electrosurgery is not a synonym for *electrocautery* but is often erroneously referred to as electrocautery in practice and literature.

PRINCIPLES OF ELECTROCAUTERY

Principles of electrocautery

Radiofrequency Generator:

- ❖ Generates high-frequency currents (100 K-Hz to 4 MHz) which induces ionic vibration but no movement.
- ❖ Ionic vibration generates intracellular heat but no muscle/nerve depolarization.
- ❖ Power settings are in Watts (amps x volts).

Intracellular heat can cause:

- ❖ boiling + explosion (CUT), and/or
- ❖ dehydration (desiccation), and/or
- ❖ fire sparks (fulguration).

Dehydration + Fire sparks = Coagulation

BLUE SIDE

- ❖ COAGULATION
- ❖ Activation: Blue Pedal
- ❖ Settings: blue side ONLY

❖ Modes: – Monopolar , A P C, Bip o l a r

❖ Outlets: separate for monopolar & bipolar

YELLOW SIDE

❖ CUT

❖ Activation: Yellow Pedal

❖ S e t t i n g s: yellow side ONLY

❖ Modes: P u r e c u t, Blend–Cut with several "modes"   with   different   "on" /" off" ratios.

❖ Outlet usually single.

Basic Physics Terminology

❖ Voltage (volts): force   that   pushes   the current ("Potential Energy"). – More force = more destruction

❖ Resistance (ohm): quality of tissue that impedes flow of current. – More resistance = less current flow. – Resistance of skin > bone > fat > muscle > bowel wall (326 ohms) > blood.

❖ Intensity (amps): amount of electricity crossing an area (wire), per second.

- ❖ Current Density (amp/cm^2): amount of current flowing through a cross sectional area = Current Intensity(amps)/area(cm^2)

Point to Remember

The amount of Energy delivered to the "active" device (snare, hot forceps, sphincterotome, etc) is the same than the delivered to the "indifferent plate", but the "current density" is very different due to the small "active" end compared with the large "indifferent plate".

Basic Physics Terminology

- ❖ Generated heat: is proportional to the square of the current density: (Intensity/area)^2.
- ❖ Small area of lesion/stalk causes disproportional high heat.
- ❖ Power output: Is given in Watts = amps x volts. Voltage is constant, hence higher output increases the intensity of current (amps).
- ❖ Higher output = higher current density = much higher heat

- ❖ Delivered Energy: Is given in Joules. Energy (watts) x time (seconds)

Types of Electrocautery

Monopolar (Needs separate "return electrode")

- o Coagulation (6% "on" duty cycle)
- o Argon Plasma (non-contact coagulation)
- o Contact coagulation

Cut

- o Pure (100% "on" duty cycle)
- o Blend (12-80% "on" duty cycle); usually 25-50%
- ❖ Bipolar (active and return electrode are side-to-side)

ERBE Electrocautery

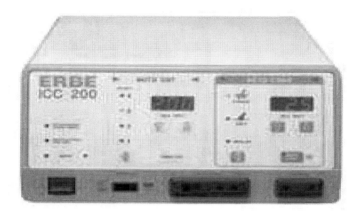

Electrocautery modes

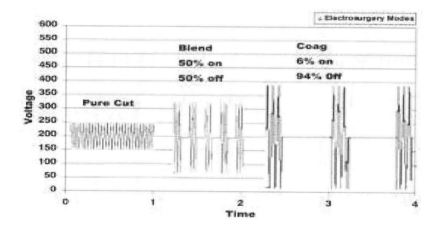

Physical Process Desiccation (Coagulation)

- ❖ Slow heating of tissue in close contact, then fluid loss with bubbling, then steam release with cooling, then restarts, slow heating of tissue in close contact, then ···
- ❖ Main Effect: Desiccation/Coagulation, with preemptive HEMOSTASIS.
- ❖ Best Instrument: – Microbipolar (no fulguration).

Alternatives:

- ❖ Monopolar coagulation @ 20-30 W, or
- ❖ Blend-cut with high-CREST (3 or more) or low % duty @ 20-40W

CONSIDERATIONS:

- ❖ If setting is too low, may desiccate too deep; difficult to cut.
- ❖ If too high and monopolar, may give deep fulguration.
- ❖ Pressing on wall increases burn depth (pull in Hot Bx.)

Physical Process Fulguration

- ❖ Electrode not in contact with tissue (or insulated by desiccated tissue): ionization of surrounding air, then long spark with high current density, then superficial coagulation, then (if you continue) deep necrosis with black eschar.
- ❖ Effect: Tissue ablation.
- ❖ Best instrument: - Argon Plasma Coagulator @ 40-60 W.

Alternative:

- ❖ Monopolar coagulation, or
- ❖ Blend-cut with high-CREST at high setting.

High risk of transmural necrosis with prolonged burn (continuous "painting" in APC); use "saline pillow".

Physical Process Cutting

- ❖ In low resistant tis sue (GI mucosa): Initial desiccation, then increased tissue resistance, then short spark, then very rapid tissue heating, then intracellular boiling, then cell explosion, then steam release, then desiccation, then increased tissue resistance, then, ...

Effect: Cut

Best instrument:

- ❖ Monopolar "pure" Cut @ high energy
- ❖ Monopolar Blend-Cut with high % "on" duty, or low CREST.

CONSIDERATIONS:

- ❖ Needs water in tissue (not completely desiccated) and loose contact (short sparks).
- ❖ Works better with high-continuous energy 60-100 Watts

Monopolar Electrocautery

Has a large "Indifferent Plate" for electricity return and a small "active electrode"; - causes high current density and very high heat at active electrode.

CAUTIONS: - Causes deeper injury, hence is bad choice to control active bleeding (high perforation risk except with noncontact technique like APC). - There must be absence of flammable gases (bowel lavage) to avoid explosion.

Indifferent plate should: - A) be near to site of active electrode, to decrease resistance from other tissues, - B) have conductive gel to decrease skin resistance, - C) remain in complete contact all the time (dual plate w monitoring circuit confirms contact) to maximize energy in active electrode.

Examples: hot snare, hot biopsy, Argon Plasma Coagulator, sphincterotome, needle knife.

Monopolar Modes: Contact Coagulation

- ❖ Very short "active" sinus wave (6-10% of cycle) with long cooling period (off, or inactive 90-94% of cycle).
- ❖ Long "cooling" facilitates desiccation, high "peak voltage" facilitates fulguration (CREST 7-8).
- ❖ Causes slow heating (excellent desiccation) followed with spark and superficial fulguration, after desiccation is complete. - Deep fulguration can give transmural necrosis

- ❖ Close contact gives more desiccation, but loose contact or complete desiccation of surrounding tissue causes more fulguration/necrosis (keep continuous close contact).
- ❖ Complication: Post-polypectomy bleed after 2-8 days.

Argon Plasma Coagulation (Non-Contact Electrocoagulation)

- ❖ Argon gas flowing inside hollow catheter and ionized by monopolar current in wire inside catheter.
- ❖ Needs "indifferent plate" and absence of flammable gases.
- ❖ Causes coagulation at point of nearest conductive (non desiccated) tissue: "around the corner" coagulation.
- ❖ Distance of probe to tissue, and length of therapy: – 2-8 mm (2-3 mm at lower setting) x 0.5-2 sec.
- ❖ Depth of injury is decreased by "saline pillow" (from 86% to 21% deep).

Power:

- For ablation, best setting is 70-90 W @ 1 LPM.

- For hemostasis , best setting is 40-50 @ 0.5 LPM; Poor hemostasis in active bleeding (dissipation).

PRECAUTIONS:

- Injury can be deep; give short bursts (tap) or continuous movement "painting" .

- Use lower setting if in contact with metal stents.

- Avoid contact (gas injection and monopolar transmural burn),

- Avoid fluid pool (energy dissipation),

- Suction between treatments to decrease gas distention/perforation risk.

Monopolar Modes Pure Cut, Blend cut

Pure Cut: 100% on continuous sinusoidal wave without cooling-off period.

❖ Causes very rapid heating with cell explosion and formation of steam and sparks.

-Gives little coagulation (no desiccation) -Current has a very low "peak voltage" /" root of mean square voltage" ratio (low CREST < 2)

-Not used in endoscopy, unless some coagulation was given first.

-Complication: immediate bleed

Blend-Cut:

Sinus wave duty cycle is "on" 25-50% of the time; allows for some cooling-off period (50-75% of time)

- Gives less cell explosion (cut) than pure-cut, and moderate desiccation + fulguration (coagulation)

- Has higher CREST than pure-cut (2.2-5)

- At same energy setting has higher peak voltage, hence can fulgurate more. - Different levels of "blend" are set by the manufacturer.

- In ERBE: Effect-1= minimal coag; Effect-4 = maximal coag; ENDO-CUT uses Effect-3 (high coag alternating with blend-cut)

- Responds only to "CUT setting"

- Loose contact facilitates "blend" process.

Complication: Post-polypectomy bleed within 12 hours.

Point to Remember

In general, at identical Power Setting (watts):

- COAGULATION currents cause deeper tissue injury than CUT (pure or blend) currents.

- HOT FORCEPS cause deeper tissue injury than HOT SNARES.

REMEMBER Yellow + Blue IS NOT Green

COAGULATION (Blue) unit is completely independent of CUT (Yellow) unit;

- Power setting in COAG side does not affect the CUT side.

BLEND-CUT current is a feature of the CUT (Yellow) unit.

- The degree of "blending" depends on the chosen mode (Endo-Cut, vs blend-1, vs blend-2, etc.)

Endoscopic Electrocoagulation Techniques

Snare Polypectomy

VARIABLES

- ❖ Energy
- ❖ Wave: coag vs blend-c
- ❖ Stalk diameter
- ❖ Wire tension (>1.5cm)
- ❖ Wire diamet(.3-.4mm)

PHASES

· Desiccation

· Cut: mechanical vs electrosurg. vs mixed

− Sequential

− Combined

Snare Polypectomy

· Desiccation: − COAG @ 20-30 (25)W, or Blend Cut 2 @ 20-30 W, or Endo-Cut-3@ 200 W; − Lower energy on Rt colon. Higher in thick stalk.

− Saline "pillow" in sessile lesions.

– Avoid:

· Too much desiccation: difficult to cut; transmural necrosis

· Polyp contact with other wall: burn (shake it)

· Fluid pool: loss of energy.

Cutting:

A) Mechanical or Mixed: close snare with constant mild-moderate pressure during or after COAGULATION.

B) Electrosurgical: Close snare with very light hold during Blend-Cut or Endo-Cut.

· If snare gets stuck after excessive desiccation, change to pure-cut @ 100-150 W. (If tissue is too dry, will not cut)

Hot Biopsy

· COAG (Fulgurate-COAG) @ 25 W, or ERBE Soft-COAG @ 60 W

– Tent-pull tissue right & left, close & away, with short "tap" to coagulate all base; do not "overcook"; then pull to remove.

- Adequate for lesions up to 5 mm (cold snare is preferred); used in difficult-to-snare position.

· Residual polyp in Cold Bx = 30% of patients

· Residual polyp in Hot Bx = 17% of patients

· Residual polyp in cold snare = rare

- Saline "pillow" has little effect in decreasing thermal injury in Hot Biopsy ("tenting" is important).

Sphincterotomy

· Endo-Cut-3 @ 200 W, or Blend-Cut 2 (medium CREST of 3) @ 40 W, or PureCut @ 30 W.

- At least 1/3 of wire outside the papillae to decrease over-coagulation and pancreatitis

- Low wire tension to prevent "Zipper"

- Blend-Cut / Endo-Cut causes less pancreatitis

Bipolar Electrocautery

· Usually gives low-energy or "micro-bipolar". Has two or more small active electrodes very close to each other (active and return electrode)

· Does not use "indifferent plate".

· Risk of explosion with flammable gases (needs colon prep)

· Less depth of injury. Saline pillow further decreases depth of injury (very important in colon & small bowel).

· Excellent desiccation and coagulation at low settings (15- 20 W). Excellent for hemostasis.

· Example: BICAP, Gold-Probe.

Micro-Bipolar Mode

· Used only for hemostasis (BICAP and GoldProbe);

- Tumor-Probe use was very limited.

· Depth of burn is limited and "saline pillow" can decrease it further.

· Better effect with large 10-Fr probes (needs "Therapeutic-channel" (T) Scope)

· Settings, pressure applied, and length of time have been standardized.

Complications of Electrocautery

· Indifferent-Plate & EKG-Pad: burn

· Fetal Stimulation

· Capacitive Coupling Discharge: burn

· Pacemaker: interference, burn, or device damage.

· Implantable Cardioverter Defibrillator: trigger, device damage, or asystole (dual system)

· Deep Brain stimulator and Gastric stimulator: "shock", burn, or device damage.

· Bowel Explosion

Complications Indifferent-Plate & EKG-Pad Burn Fetal Stimulation

· Skin burn from Indifferent Plate (Return Electrode):

36

- If partial detachment causes small contact area, and high current density, giving a burn.

· EKG electrode pad burn: — If indifferent plate is separated, and EKG pads acts as "indifferent plate"; EKG electrodes should be > 0.3 cm2 each

· Fetal Stimulation: — if electricity passes through the uterus to reach "indifferent-plate"

· Prevention: — Dual-Pad with "Return electrode Monitor" (REM) circuit, detects change in surface/resistance and "shuts-off" the unit.

— During pregnancy, indifferent-plate should not be placed causing the uterus to be between electrode & plate.

Complications Capacitive Coupling Discharge

· Scope works as capacitor of currents induced by snare/hot-forceps;

— important only with large scopes (Colon/ERCP).

· Scope can discharge current after contact with "frame-wires" (damaged external surface) or eye piece; can burn physician or inside of patient.

Prevention:

- S-cord connects "scope frame" to "indifferent plate" and unloads charge.

- Risk: if indifferent plate gets off, scope acts as indifferent plate; should be used with "dual-pad" /REM.

Complications Pacemaker Interference

· Electrocautery generates electromagnetic fields of up to 60 V/m

· Pacemakers are inhibited with electromagnetic fields > 0.1 V/m.

· Permanent protective circuit may be damaged or need reprogramming if current is delivered close to pacemaker or its leads.

· With poorly grounded or non-isolated electrocautery, pacemaker can work as "indifferent plate" and cause myocardial burn or arrhythmia (use "dual-pads").

RECOMMENDATION Pacemaker Interference

RECOMMENDATION:

- "Pacemaker-dependent" for rhythm or hemodynamics (20%): use magnet

· pacemaker should be placed on " continuous asynchronous pacing" (VOO or DOO) with a "ring magnet", only while only while electrocautery current is delivered. electrocautery current is delivered.

· after electrocoagulation, the pacemaker should be reactivated and assessed for normal function (telephonically).

- "No pacemaker-dependent" : magnet use is optional

· used mostly for prolonged electrocautery use, like in APC for GAVE or radiation proctitis.

Complications   Implantable   Cardioverter Defibrillator

· Damage can occur as in case of pacemakers

· Electrocautery waves can be interpreted as "R waves" simulating arrhythmia or normal rhytm, and ICD will respond cardioverting, or inhibiting cardioversion or pacing.

· Most, but not all, ICDs respond to properly placed "magnet" by "suspension of tachycardia detection", and/or "suspension of ICD therapy", without affecting pacemaker function.

Complications Implantable Cardioverter Defibrillator

· Patient with ICD who is "pacemaker dependent" will not have pacer changed to "asynchronous pacing" by the magnet:

- Risk of prolonged pacemaker inhibition by electrocautery, with asystole.

· Is difficult to ascertain if magnet is properly placed over ICD;

- Change in position may affect inhibition.

· Is difficult to know beforehand which effect magnet will have on the ICD.

- Example: ICDs made by "Guidant" may respond to magnet by:

1) Permanent disabling ICD therapy,

2) Temporary disabling ICD therapy, or

3) No change at all

Non-Electrocautery Thermal Device

Thermocoagulation Heater Probe

· Can irrigate and tamponade + coagulate.

· Can be applied "en face" or "tangential".

· 10 Fr probe is better, but needs "T-channel scope".

· Is not electrocautery (no sparks); safe in unprepared bowel.

· Has an electrically heated coil inside a Teflon-covered insulated cylinder; heats to 110 oC degrees.

· Power setting in Joules (Watts x sec): HP unit decides time needed to deliver the requested energy.

· In ulcer; apply in 4 quadrants plus center.

CHEMICAL CAUTERY

Chemical cautery

Many chemical reactions can destroy tissue and some are used routinely in medicine, most commonly for the removal of small skin lesions (i.e. warts or necrotized tissue) or hemostasis. The disadvantages are that chemicals can leach into areas where cauterization was not intended. For this reason, laser and electrical methods are preferable, where practical. Some cauterizing agents are:

❖ Silver nitrate: Active ingredient of the lunar caustic, a stick that traditionally looks like a large match-stick. It is dipped into water and pressed onto the lesion to be cauterized for a few moments.

❖ Trichloroacetic acid

❖ Cantharidin: An extract of the blister beetle that causes epidermal necrosis and blistering; used to treat warts.

Nasal cauterization

If a person has been having frequent nose bleeds, it is most likely caused by an exposed blood vessel in their nose. Even if the nose is not bleeding at the time, it is cauterized to prevent future bleeding. The different methods of cauterization include burning the affected area with acid, hot metal, lasers, or silver nitrate. Such a procedure is naturally quite painful. Sometimes liquid nitrogen is used as a less painful alternative, though it is less effective. In the few countries that permit the use of cocaine for medicinal purposes, it is occasionally used topically to make this procedure less uncomfortable, cocaine being the only local anesthetic which also produces vasoconstriction, making it ideal for controlling nosebleeds.

INDICATIONS OF ELECTROCAUTERY

Aims and objectives

❖ Prevent or stop bleeding after an injury or during surgery

❖ Remove abnormal tissue growth

❖ Prevent infection

Basically, the purpose of cautery is to destroy tissue. The burns produced are typically second degree (blisters), but if handled clumsily can easily become third degree burns that go clear through the skin.

Surgical cautery is often used in modern settings to seal a single stubborn blood vessel, to carefully pare off or to destroy unwanted tissue as in the case of cancerous cells, moles, or lesions caused by viruses, or to surgically separate tissues with minimal blood loss. The two types of cautery used for modern surgical intervention include electrocautery which uses an electrical instrument to generate the burns or chemical cautery which involves the application of acids, freezing chemicals, or other chemical substances that produce a chemical or frost burn.

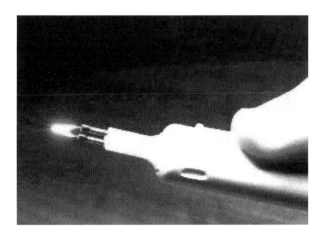

Electrical instrument for electrocautery

INDICATIONS OF ELECTROCAUTERY

Electrocautery is a safe and effective method of hemostasis during cutaneous surgery. It is also useful in the treatment of various small benign skin lesions, although only lesions that do not require histological review should be treated with electrocautery.

Electrocautery shares many indications with electrosurgery and is of particular importance in patients who have implanted electrical devices in whom external electromagnetic interference should be avoided. Furthermore, unlike electrosurgical instruments, electrocautery devices maintain function in a wet field. The treatment has a number of uses:

Surgery

A surgeon may use this technique to cut through soft tissue during surgery so they can gain access to a site on the body they need to get to. Electrocauterization allows the surgeon to seal off blood vessels that are bleeding during surgery. Sealing off blood vessels helps prevent blood loss and keeps the site clean.

Tumor Removal

This method is sometimes used to remove abnormal tissue growth such as tumors. This approach is common for growths located in sensitive or areas that are difficult to reach, such as the brain.

46

Nasal Treatment

If get frequent nosebleeds, it's likely an exposed blood vessel in nose is causing them. Doctor may recommend this type of treatment even if nose is not bleeding at the time you seek medical advice.

Wart Removal

This technique is frequently used to treat genital warts or warts on other areas of the body. Wart removal usually only requires one treatment.

Low temperatures can be used for superficial tissue destruction in the treatment of superficial and relatively avascular lesions, including the following:

- ❖ Seborrheic keratoses
- ❖ Acrochordons
- ❖ Molluscum
- ❖ Verrucae
- ❖ Syringomas
- ❖ Small angiomas

A dermal curette may be used concurrently to remove the lesion. Higher temperatures are effective in removing thicker skin lesions, such as the following:

- ❖ Sebaceous hyperplasia
- ❖ Pyogenic granulomas
- ❖ Hemostasis of vessels in surgery

Other indications for electrocautery include the following:

- ❖ Vasectomy
- ❖ Punctual occlusion (for dry eye syndrome)

PREOPERATIVE CARE FOR TREATMENT

Preoperative care

Preoperative care for electrocautery involves identifying and eliminating potential safety hazards to the patient and operating team. A thorough patient history and physical should be performed to determine the patient's general medical condition; to identify any risk factors for excessive bleeding, susceptibility to infection, or poor wound healing; and to note any allergies to antiseptics, anesthetics, and dressings, among others.

The treatment team wears gloves and masks, and smoke-evacuation equipment should be available. The lesion and the area surrounding are cleaned with nonalcohol solution such as chlorhexidine or povidone iodine. For malignant lesions, marking the clinical border of the tumor may be useful, as anesthetics can blur the margins. If alcohol is used, ensure that the area is dry before beginning the procedure.

Local injection of 1% lidocaine is typically used prior to in-office procedures. Lidocaine with epinephrine can be used for vasoconstrictive effects if injected 15 minutes prior to the start of the procedure. Depending on the tolerance of the patient, some procedures, such as removal of acrochordons or small angiomas, do not require anesthesia. Alternatively, instead of lidocaine, liquid nitrogen can be used as cryoanesthesia prior to procedures.

Equipment includes but is not limited to the following:

- Surgical mask with eye protection
- Gloves
- Antiseptic solution
- Fenestrated drape
- Lidocaine 1% with or without epinephrine
- Syringe
- Injection needles
- Gauze, 4 x 4 inch
- Dental rolls

- ❖ Electrocautery (thermal cautery) unit/disposable pen
- ❖ Electrode tips
- ❖ Sterile hand sheath
- ❖ Smoke evacuator
- ❖ Marking pen

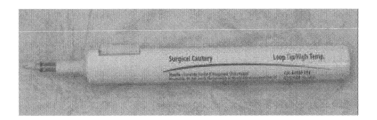

Electrocautery device

Electrocautery devices can be in the form of disposable battery-powered pens or line-powered thermal cautery units.

Disposable Electrosurgical Pencil, 4mm Banana Connector

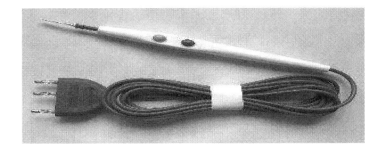

Electro Cauterization of Skin Tags: Advantages and Disadvantages

Electro cauterization is a process in which an instrument is heated electrically and then applied to the skin tag to burn its cells. The process is conducted by a qualified and trained health professional. It usually involves the following steps.

1. The area is cleaned throughout
2. The area is numbed by means of local anesthetic.
3. The needle is heated and then put over the skin tag
4. The contact of the needle with the tag burns its cell.
5. The burnt cells are then removed from the area.
6. Some doctors would like to send a specimen of the cells to the lab.
7. A bandage is applied around the treated area.

Advantages

1. Quick fix method. It is quick. A normal skin tags treatment takes around 20 minutes. So you are tag free within 20 minutes.

2. Less Expensive. It has been found that electro-cauterization is less expensive as compared to other surgical methods such as cryosurgery and laser therapy.

3. One session is usually enough. In case of cryosurgery and laser therapy you may need to pay several visits to the clinic. On the other hand, in electro-cauterization, it is a one off thing in most cases.

Disadvantages

1. It is invasive.

2. It is not pain free. It may be painful during and after the treatment. Post-treatment pain generally continues for a few days.

3. Healing times. It takes less time to burn it but it takes a lot longer for the wound to heal. Also anti-biotic are no good for

general health and immune system.

4. No good for a large number. Although it is a quick method for a tag or two, but what if you have mor? Sometimes people may have, 5, 10, 20 or even more tags on their body. It will take a lot of time, money and effort to remove them this way. The post-treatment pain in this case is horrible.

APPROACH CONSIDERATIONS

Approach Considerations

In addition to hemostasis, achieved by direct contact of the electrode tip to the damaged vessel, electrocautery can be used in various procedures. Detailed descriptions of a few electrocautery procedures are described below:

Pinpoint cautery

❖ Spider angiomas are superficial vascular lesions composed of small veins that radiate from a central dilated arteriole. The pinpoint cautery technique can be used to treat superficial telangiectasias such as this.

❖ The lesion is cleaned with nonalcohol antiseptic solution.

❖ Anesthetic is not necessary for this procedure.

❖ A glass slide is placed on the lesion with pressure to locate the feeding vessel.

- ❖ A fine needle electrode tip is used in the electrocautery device.
- ❖ The cold needle is placed into the lesion and current is applied for less than 1 second.
- ❖ The scab that develops will fall off within 10 days.

Removal of Small Benign Lesions

Small benign lesions such as acrochordons, seborrheic keratoses, and molluscum can be removed in the manner below.

- ❖ The lesion is cleaned and area anesthetized.
- ❖ A pinpoint or ballpoint electrode tip is touched directly to the lesion.
- ❖ The electrode should be inactivated once the lesion appears to become necrotic or separates from the dermis.
- ❖ The lesion will fall off within 10 days, or a curette or gauze may be used to remove abnormal tissue.
- ❖ Larger, more exophytic lesions can be shaved flat prior to electrocautery of the base.

- ❖ Benign lesions can be removed until the surface of the skin appears flat with normal contours to avoid scarring and ensure good cosmesis.
- ❖ For highly vascular lesions such as pyogenic granuloma, the lesion is injected using 1% lidocaine with epinephrine 15 minutes prior to the start of the procedure, allowing vasoconstriction to take full effect.

Surgical Punctal Occlusion

- ❖ Punctal occlusion surgery is used in patients with severe dry eye disease who experience recurrent punctual plug extrusions or punctual plug complications.
- ❖ The area is cleaned and anesthetized using an infratrochlear nerve block with lidocaine.
- ❖ A high-temperature electrocautery device with a fine tip is inserted cold into the lacrimal punctum, the vertical portion of lacrimal canaliculus, and the horizontal portion of lacrimal canaliculus.

- ❖ The device is then turned on until the surrounding punctual tissue becomes white (10-14 seconds).
- ❖ The device is then removed slowly and antibiotic ointment is applied.

PATIENTS EDUCATION AND CONSENT

The steps, risks, benefits, possible complications, and alternatives of electrocautery should be explained to the patient. Consent from the patient or a legal patient representative must be obtained prior to the procedure.

Contraindications

There are no absolute contraindications to electrocautery.

Technical Considerations

Each electrocautery device can deliver heat at a single temperature or range of temperatures, between 100o C and 1200o C. Most devices also include interchangeable tips such as loops, fine tips, and needle tips.

Physicians must consider the histologic properties of the tissue to be treated, the area and depth of destruction desired, possible complications, and capabilities of the different electrocautery devices. A common principle of all electrosurgical procedures is to use the least amount of power possible to achieve the desired effect, limiting damage to the adjacent tissue.

Risks

Risks of electrocautery are:

- ❖ Bleeding. Blood loss is usually minimal, because the electrocautery seals blood vessels as it removes warts.
- ❖ Infection. Antibiotics may be given at the time of the procedure to reduce the risk of infection.
- ❖ Pain. Medicine may be needed for several days after the electrocautery procedure.

COMPLICATIONS PREVENTION

As with any procedure, there are potential risks to the patient, as well as the operating physician.

Burns

There is a risk of fire or explosion if flammable materials are in close proximity to the treatment site. Alcohol, oxygen, and bowel gas are all highly flammable. Alcohol cleansers should be avoided; if they are used, they should be allowed to dry completely. If the patient uses a portable oxygen generator, it should be stopped briefly for the procedure. Eschar buildup should be removed from the surgical electrode to avoid sparking or flaming.

Transmission of infection

The same principles of infection transmission apply to both electrosurgery and electrocautery. The 3 potential modes for infection transmission in these procedures include the treatment electrode, surgical smoke, and aerosolized blood microdroplets. Experimental studies involving animal skin have shown transmission of hepatitis B virus, human papillomavirus (HPV), and Staphylococcus aureus from an inoculated site to an uninfected site by means of the contaminated electrodesiccation electrode.

During electrosurgical procedures, aerosolized blood droplets can be propelled a distance of up to 30 cm and can be infectious if inhaled. Surgical smoke can also contain viable viruses and bacteria, in addition to hazardous chemicals and carcinogens. Viable HPV virus has been identified in the vapor of warts being treated with electrocoagulation.

To prevent the risks of infection transmission, a smoke-evacuating system should be used, along with facial masks, protective eye wear, and surgical gloves. Disposable or sterilized electrodes should be used.

CHEMICAL CAUTERY

Chemical cautery is one of two forms of cauterization, the medical term applied to destroying tissue or clotting blood by closing off a part of the body with heat, cold, or caustic substance. This form is cauterization with a chemical agent, while the other main type, electrocautery, is cauterization by electricity.

Chemical cautery is a technique of applying caustic chemicals such as Trichloroacetic acid (TCA), Glycolic acid, Phenol, Silver nitrate, Sodium hydroxide to remove various skin growths such as skin tags, warts, corns, molluscum contagiosum. The chemicals are used at various strengths depending on the type and site of the lesions and it can be done at multiple sittings.

Chemical cautery was developed in the early 20th century as a sinus treatment, chemical cautery is commonly used to perform simple medical procedures that relieve common ailments. Examples include wart removal, treatment of ingrown nails, as well as treatment for sinus problems. It is an in-office procedure, and in the case of relief for sinus pain sufferers, is typically quite simple and painless.

To relieve sinus pain, a medical professional uses chemicals to destroy the mast cells in the sinus cavities that release histamine and other sources of inflammation that leads to sinus pain. Not all patients suffering from sinus pain are eligible for this type of cautery, but those with recurring symptoms that persist in spite of anti-histamine and other drugs are typical candidates. The procedure takes about 15 to 20 minutes and often has to be repeated a few times each year.

Chemical cautery is also used in dermatology to destroy unhealthy skin tissue. Though cryotherapy is sometimes used as a treatment for warts, other forms of cautery can also be effective. Dermatologists, ear nose and throat specialists, dentists, and some family doctors and internists often offer these treatments in their office.

Agents that act as a chemical cautery include phenol, silver nitrate, and liquid nitrogen. Some of these are readily available and can be handy for pet owners as well as people. It is the same principal applied when using styptic powder on pet nails that bleed if trimmed to short. Silver nitrate is also an effective treatment for canker sores or mouth ulcers.

FREQUENTLY ASKED QUESTIONS

FREQUENTLY ASKED QUESTIONS (FAQ'S)

WHAT IS ELECTROCAUTERY (EC)?

Electrocautery is a method using electricity for removal of various unwanted skin lesions. A very mild strength of electricity is used to heat the needle which will cut out lesions from the surface of the skin.

WHICH SKIN LESIONS CAN BE REMOVED WITH EC?

Electrocautery is commonly used to remove benign lesions on the surface of the skin such as warts, skin tags and seborrheic keratosis. It can also be used to control bleeding on the surface of the skin following shave biopsy or curettage.

WHAT HAPPENS WHEN YOU GET YOUR NOSE CAUTERIZED?

If the source of the bleeding is a blood vessel that is easily seen, a doctor may cauterize it (seal the blood vessel) with a chemical called silver nitrate.

Cauterization is most effective when the bleeding is coming from the very front part of the nose.

WHAT DOES THE PROCEDURE INVOLVE?

The procedure is very simple and takes less than 20 minutes. The lesion and the area around the skin will be numbed with local anaesthesia which will cause a slight discomfort. After few second a tool with a needle tip is used to cut out the lesion from the skin. The tool can also be used to stop any bleeding on the surface of the skin following the procedure. After the procedure, the wound is covered with a small bandage. You will be given information on wound care by the team.

WHAT IS THE AVERAGE TIME FOR SCARS TO HEAL AFTER ELECTROCAUTERY?

It normally takes 1-2 weeks for spots to heal after electrocautery treatment. It's important to use sun protection to optimize healing.

WHY IT IS DONE?

Electrocautery removes warts with little blood loss. It usually is used for small areas of warts.

WHAT TO EXPECT AFTER CAUTERY

The recovery time depends on the location and number of warts removed.

- ❖ After cautery you may have some pain, swelling, and redness.
- ❖ Healing usually occurs within 2 to 4 weeks.
- ❖ Healing time may be prolonged if a large area of tissue is burned.
- ❖ Scarring may occur.

WHAT ARE THE SIDE EFFECTS WITH EC?

Mild pain during the local anesthesia injection is common. Rarely, bleeding during the procedure can occur. However, it can easily be controlled with compression. You should not forget to inform your doctor, if you are on blood-thinning agents such as aspirin or warfarin.

What is chemical cautery therapy?

Chemical cautery therapy is a painless, office-based, non-invasive treatment for a wide variety of sinus problems. It was initially developed at the

University of Iowa and has been used in several other ENT practices in the Midwest.

The chemical cautery treatment process is a non-invasive approach to managing chronic sinus problems. It involves a series of treatments over time (usually 2-3 treatments per year) to maintain long-lasting relief from symptoms and protection from infections. Chemical cautery frequently takes the place of other medications, in some cases eliminating the need for antihistamines, decongestants, and nasal sprays. This makes it a very cost-effective and time efficient treatment.

Doesn't "cautery" mean the nose is being damaged or burnt?

Chemical cautery does not burn the nasal lining tissue and causes no lasting harm. It is not a treatment to stop a nosebleed.

Does chemical cautery hurt?

No. The treatment is mildly irritating to the lining of the nose for about one hour after treatment. This promotes clearing of the sinuses.

Once this initial effect has passed, there is no discomfort whatsoever.

Does chemical cautery damage the nasal lining?

No. Chemical cautery has been used for decades, and no complications have been reported. The medications used are very mild and cannot injure the nasal lining.

What is involved in starting chemical cautery?

Chemical cautery involves a series of three sprays of medications to the nasal airways after first decongesting the nose with a powerful decongestant. The entire treatment takes about 5 minutes. Treatments are spaced out. To start the chemical cautery therapy, patients undergo monthly treatments for three months. Over time, the effect wears off, so booster treatments are given about every four to six months.

How does chemical cautery work?

Doctors believe that chemical cautery works by improving the self-cleaning properties of the nasal and sinus lining. If the entire lining of the nose were laid out flat, it would be the size of an unfolded newspaper. That's big surface area to interact with germs, pollen, and irritants.

The body protects the nose's lining with a sophisticated cleaning system. Under a microscope, the nose's lining looks like shag carpet. Each fiber represents a cilia, which is basically a brush. Each of these cilia move about 800 times each minute to constantly sweep a thin layer of protective mucous across the lining of the nose like a giant conveyor belt or a moving carpet.

When germs, pollen, or irritants get trapped in the mucous, the healthy nose quickly sweeps the problem away. In the diseased nose, the mucous does not flow normally. When germs, pollen, or irritants land on the nasal lining, they sit there and gum things up. This triggers inflammation and can cause or maintain sinusitis. By re-establishing the self-cleaning properties of the nose, chemical cautery reverses and prevents a wide variety of sinus problems.

Who is a candidate for chemical cautery?

Many sinus sufferers will benefit from chemical cautery. It is generally helpful for:

- ❖ Sinus infections
- ❖ Allergies
- ❖ Sinus headaches
- ❖ Facial pain
- ❖ Facial pressure
- ❖ Nasal congestion
- ❖ Nasal stuffiness
- ❖ Ear pressure and recurrent ear infections

How do I know if I am a candidate for chemical cautery?

If you have any of the symptoms listed above or if you consider yourself to be a "sinus sufferer," you are a candidate for chemical cautery. You should be seen by your physicians for assessment and diagnosis.

Does chemical cautery work for everyone?

Roughly 80% of chemical cautery patients who are felt to be candidates by physicians will do very well with Chemical Cautery. For some patients, after careful assessment, Chemical Cautery is not the right method of treatment. In virtually every case, however, our physicians can provide relief through other interventions.

How will I know if chemical cautery is helping me?

Most patients will notice a difference after 2 treatments. For patients who have convincing improvement in their symptoms, chemical cautery will be a good long-term treatment method.

Are the effects of chemical cautery permanent?

No. Booster treatments are required – usually every 4-6 months. It is very common for doctors to hear, "I could tell it was time for a treatment…" at the 4-6 month booster treatment visit.

REFERENCES

REFERENCES

1. "Dictionary definition, retrieved: 2016-03-07."
   http://dictionary.reference.com/browse/cautery

2. Robinson, Victor, Ph.C., M.D. (editor) (1939). "Actual cautery". The Modern Home Physician, A New Encyclopedia of Medical Knowledge. WM. H. Wise & Company (New York)., page 16.

3. The Presocratic Influence upon Hippocratic Medicine

4. Surgical Instruments from Ancient Rome (hsl.virginia.edu/historical/artifacts/romal) retrieved on dated 29.03.16

5. Mohamed Kamel Hussein (1978), The Concise History of Medicine and Pharmacy (cf. Mostafa Shehata, "The Father Of Islamic Medicine: An International Questionnaire", Journal of the

International Society for the History of Islamic Medicine, 2002 (2): 58-59 [58])

6. R McElroy for details of various operations and the unintended effects of chemical cauterization.

7. Sabiston textbook of surgery (19th ed.). 2012. p. 235

8. Soon SL, Washington CV. Electrosurgery, electrocoagulation, electrodesiccation, electrofulguration, electrosection, electrocautery. Robinson JK, Hanke CW, Siegel DM, et al. *Surgery of the Skin.* 2nd edition. Elsevier; 2010. Ch 9.

9. Lane JE, O'brien EM, Kent DE. Optimization of thermocautery in excisional dermatologic surgery. *Dermatol Surg.* 2006 May. 32(5):669-75.

10. Hainer BL. Electrosurgery for the skin. *Am Fam Physician.* 2002 Oct 1. 66(7):1259-66

11. Laughlin SA, Dudley DK. Electrosurgery. *Clin Dermatol.* 1992 Jul-Sep. 10(3):285-90.

12. Labrecque M, Nazerali H, Mondor M, Fortin V, Nasution M. Effectiveness and complications associated with 2 vasectomy occlusion techniques. *J Urol.* 2002 Dec. 168(6):2495-8; discussion 2498.

13. Schmidt SS, Minckler TM. The vas after vasectomy: comparison of cauterization methods. *Urology.* 1992 Nov. 40(5):468-70

14. Hutnik CM, Probst LE. Argon laser punctal therapy versus thermal cautery for the treatment of aqueous deficiency dry eye syndrome. *Can J Ophthalmol.* 1998 Dec. 33(7):365-72.

15. Harris DW. ABC of dermatology. Procedures. *Br Med J (Clin Res Ed).* 1988 Mar 12. 296(6624):769-71.

16. Spiller WF, Spiller RF. Cryoanesthesia and electrosurgical treatment of benign skin tumors. *Cutis.* 1985 Jun. 35(6):551-2.

Made in the USA
Columbia, SC
16 October 2020

22990871R00041